Anilú Same Cavalcanti Ono
Shohreh Taghavaeearaby
Sonia B. Sanches

Benefits of massage therapy for Parkinson's patients

Anilú Same Cavalcanti Ono
Shohreh Taghavaeearaby
Sonia B. Sanches

Benefits of massage therapy for Parkinson's patients

And its effects on quality of life

ScienciaScripts

Imprint

Any brand names and product names mentioned in this book are subject to trademark, brand or patent protection and are trademarks or registered trademarks of their respective holders. The use of brand names, product names, common names, trade names, product descriptions etc. even without a particular marking in this work is in no way to be construed to mean that such names may be regarded as unrestricted in respect of trademark and brand protection legislation and could thus be used by anyone.

Cover image: www.ingimage.com

This book is a translation from the original published under ISBN 978-613-9-75356-7.

Publisher:
Sciencia Scripts
is a trademark of
Dodo Books Indian Ocean Ltd. and OmniScriptum S.R.L publishing group

120 High Road, East Finchley, London, N2 9ED, United Kingdom
Str. Armeneasca 28/1, office 1, Chisinau MD-2012, Republic of Moldova, Europe
Printed at: see last page
ISBN: 978-620-6-50457-3

We dedicate this Final Year Programme to our families, our dear patients and the esteemed teachers who accompanied us in our training as massage therapists.

ACKNOWLEDGEMENTS

Thanks to the Universe for the beautiful partnership that was established between us for the development of this project.

To the **great friends we made** during the fantastic journey we experienced on the Massage Therapy course.

To dear Professor **Ana Carolina de Athayde Raimundi Braz,** for her commitment to us, for her co-operation, dedication and active and affectionate participation throughout the process of building this study.

To **Dina Yasue Kagueyama Lermen** for her help and patience with our constant presence in the Library during our research times.

To our supervisor **Tatiane Romanini Gomes de Alencar.**

And to our dear patients who are the objects of this study: for their availability and willingness to embrace us in this endeavour, for their fundamental importance in the construction of this study and for our personal and professional growth.

We feel immensely honoured to have had the opportunity to meet you in this life... may we all fulfil our purposes with even more love, peace, wisdom and joy.

"Know all the theories, master all the techniques, but when you touch a human soul, be another human soul" (Cari Gustav Jung)

SUMMARY

Parkinson's Disease is characterised as a neurological disorder caused by the degeneration and death of the nerve cells of dopamine-producing neurons. It is a degenerative, chronic and progressive disease because it causes the loss of neurons in the Central Nervous System. There are many symptoms, including non-specific pain, weakness and fatigue, resting tremors, difficulty moving, muscle stiffness, loss of balance and more. Massage therapy can be used systematically to help reduce muscle tension, improve blood circulation and tissue nutrition, as well as causing physical and mental relaxation. With this in mind, the general aim of this study was to identify the benefits of massage therapy for people with Parkinson's disease, with a view to improving these symptoms. Six participants underwent 10 sessions of the technique, once a week, lasting one hour and ten minutes, at the Massage Therapy laboratory of the Federal Institute of Paraná - Londrina Campus. After the initial interview and confirmation of the diagnosis of the disease, the study's inclusion and exclusion criteria were checked before the sessions began. Participants were interviewed at the end of treatment to analyse the effects of the study. Important results were demonstrated through reports of the benefits and improvement of all participants' symptoms: muscle stiffness, tremors, non-specific pain, anxiety, sleep disturbances and constipation. The results show that massage therapy goes beyond the physical benefits, as it affects the general, psychological and emotional well-being of people with Parkinson's disease, and should be used as an adjunct to drug treatment in all cases of the disease.

Key words: massage, Parkinson's disease, benefits.

TABLE OF CONTENTS:

CHAPTER 1

1 INTRODUCTION

Parkinson's Disease is characterised as a neurological disorder caused by the degeneration and death of the nerve cells of dopamine-producing neurons. It is a degenerative, chronic and progressive disease because it causes the loss of neurons in the Central Nervous System (WERNER, 2005). Two hundred years have passed since the physician James Parkinson (1755-1824) first observed and reported cases of people walking the streets of London with a strange paralysis that hindered movement and walking, which he called agitated paralysis. It wasn't until fifty years later in Paris that neurologist Dr Jean-Martin Charcot named it Parkinson's disease in honour of Dr James Parkinson (TUMA, 2017).

Currently, according to Dr Tuma (2017), even with the surprising development of medicine in genetic and molecular research, the most advanced technology has still not managed to identify the causes of the second most common degenerative disease that causes so much suffering and weakness in its sufferers. This is a form of a disease whose causes are still unknown (idiopathic), which affects people after the age of 50 or 60, although medicine has recorded increasingly frequent cases in younger patients. It occurs more often in men, although women are also carriers, but to a lesser extent (WOOTEN, 2004).

The symptoms of Parkinson's disease are many and are divided into primary and secondary. Primary symptoms include non-specific pain, weakness and fatigue, resting tremors, difficulty moving, muscle stiffness, loss of balance and poor postural reflexes. Secondary symptoms include changes in writing and speech, sleep disorders, depression and mental degeneration (WERNER, 2005). It is known that diagnosing Parkinson's Disease is not easy, but once it has been diagnosed and drug treatment has begun, usually with Levodopa, it is important that alternative therapies or methods are incorporated into the patient's routine in order to improve their quality of life and alleviate symptoms; relaxing massage is one of the best therapies for this (quoted in PARKINSON, 2016).

Relaxing the muscles, reducing their rigidity, sharpening the senses, increasing self-esteem, sociability, combating psychological and emotional states and inducing tranquillity are some of the benefits provided by relaxation after a massage session (CASSAR, 2001).

Considering this context, the study sought to ascertain whether significant changes are achieved by sufferers of the disease in terms of reducing the symptoms manifested by the pathology. It also sought to identify the main symptoms reported by patients, as well as the benefits obtained by them in terms of improving their quality of life after receiving massage sessions, in a general context.

CHAPTER 2

2 OBJECTIVES

1.1 GENERAL OBJECTIVE:

To identify the benefits of massage therapy for people with Parkinson's disease.

1.2 SPECIFIC OBJECTIVES:

-Check the main symptoms reported by Parkinson's patients;

-To check whether the massage resulted in a reduction in the main symptoms observed in the patients;

CHAPTER 3

3 THEORETICAL BACKGROUND

This chapter was divided into parts: the first explained what Parkinson's Disease is and its symptoms. The second part explains its diagnosis and treatment. The third part deals with the fundamentals of massage therapy and pain, followed by the fourth part, which establishes the relationship between massage therapy and Parkinson's Disease, the support for this study.

3.1 PARKINSON'S DISEASE AND ITS SYMPTOMS

Parkinson's disease was first described in 1817 by the English physician James Parkinson. It is characterised as a neurological disorder caused by the degeneration of nerve cells in the so-called "substantia nigra" located in the brain. It is a degenerative disease characterised by the chronic and progressive loss of neurons in the Central Nervous System, in which there is cell death of the dopamine-producing neurons in the basal ganglia, which control and adjust the transmission of conscious commands from the cerebral cortex to the muscles of the human body (WERNER, 2005).

Parkinson's disease is debilitating, degenerative and still has no cure. Its symptoms can progress faster or slower as each individual is unique. There is no pattern to the progression of the disease (VERSAGI, 2015).

According to Sabino (2012), it is an idiopathic, primary disease of obscure cause, usually beginning after the age of 50. It is one of the most common neurological diseases, with a prevalence of between 80 and 160 cases per 100,000 inhabitants, affecting approximately 1% of people over the age of 65. Researchers at the University of Virginia Health System found that men are more likely to develop Parkinson's disease. The propensity is 1.5 times higher in men. In the study, the researchers analysed people from China, Spain, the United States, Finland, Italy and Poland.

The reasons why men are the most affected are still unknown, but what probably explains the lower incidence in women is the presence of oestrogen in the female organism, which acts as a protective factor in the nervous system (WOOTEN, 2004).

For his part, Andrade (quoted in PARKINSON, 2016) states that there is no evidence that the disease affects more men than women and that although articles on the subject have been published, scientists have not yet been able to identify the reason that triggers the development of Parkinson's Disease and that there are assumptions and hypotheses such as: the influence of toxic agents (the pesticide benomyl, a fungicide in Brazil), hormonal differences, tranquillisers, antidepressants, antivertigines, drug use (heroin), head trauma, cerebral ischaemia, viral encephalitis and genetic factors.

Parkinson's disease has primary and secondary symptoms. The primary symptoms are due to the disease itself and the secondary symptoms are a direct result of the primary symptoms. Primary symptoms are: non-specific pain, weakness and fatigue, resting tremors, bradykinesia (difficulty starting or continuing a movement), muscle rigidity and poor postural reflexes and loss of

6

balance. Secondary symptoms are related to changes in speech, staggering gait (difficulty bending arms and legs), changes in writing, sleep disturbances, depression and mental degeneration (memory loss) (WERNER, 2005).

When the neurons in the brain's substantia nigra begin to die, the amount of dopamine is reduced and generates different symptoms, including alterations in the motor system. This neurotransmitter is also responsible for memory, sleep, mood, attention and learning (quoted in PARKINSON, 2016).

The neurological alteration in the motor system is characterised by tremor that affects the fingers or hands, the head, the chin, the feet and can occur on only one side of the body or both, as well as being more intense on one side. The tremor may or may not occur when the body is stationary and not moving (rest tremor) and varies in intensity during the day (CAMBIER, MASSON, DEHEN, 1988).

According to Silva (quoted in PARKINSON, 2016), tremor is not the only manifestation of the disease. Some subtle changes can indicate that something in the body isn't right and often go unnoticed, such as: loss of smell, fixed gaze, reduction in letter size, slowness of voluntary gestures, muscle rigidity, "frozen" facial expression, tiredness, unexplained sadness, speech in a monotonous tone.

Braga *et al* (2013) states that constipation is also one of the symptoms present in Parkinson's patients and is a frequent complaint because it causes great discomfort.

3.2 DIAGNOSIS AND TREATMENT

According to Silva (cited in PARKINSON, 2016) and Moreira *et al* (2007), the diagnosis of Parkinson's disease is based on clinical criteria where the doctor, usually a neurologist in his own office, carefully analyses the patient's history, the reported symptoms and carries out a thorough physical and behavioural assessment. The doctor may order tests such as a computerised tomography scan and an encephalogram. If there are no alterations in the tests, the diagnosis of Parkinson's is confirmed. The tests are usually ordered so that the doctor can rule out other degenerative diseases.

Ferraz (2011) reports that it is not easy to diagnose Parkinson's disease and that it is necessary to pay attention to the signs and symptoms that help the doctor in his clinical diagnosis. These are: altered axial posture, difficulty turning in bed, flexed posture, reduction in the size of handwriting (micrographia), dystonia of the foot and hallux, masked face (amimia), monotonous speech, reduced blinking of the eyes or repetitive and involuntary movement of the eyelid (blepharospasm), difficulty swallowing (dysphagia), sleep disturbance, sexual disturbances, seborrhoeic dermatitis, constipation. The four cardinal signs observed are: resting tremor, rigidity, bradykinesia (abnormal slowness of voluntary movements) and decreased postural reflexes. If there is a combination of three of the four symptoms or cardinal signs or a combination of two cardinal signs, including disturbances in postural reflexes, the diagnosis of Parkinson's is clinically defined.

After being diagnosed with Parkinson's Disease, drug treatment begins. Currently, the most effective in relieving symptoms is Levodopa, a substance that is a precursor to dopamine and increases the levels of neurotransmitters in the brain. However, it is not always administered at the outset, and is usually prescribed in the more critical stages of the disease. In the early stages, Amantadine can be prescribed, an antiviral discovered as an antiparkinsonian, with more moderate actions than Levodopa and which presents itself as an alternative to drug treatment (quoted in PARKINSON, 2016).

Once the diagnosis has been made and treatment with medication has begun, it is important that alternative therapies are incorporated into the patient's routine to improve their physical and emotional quality of life. Stimulating the muscles by reducing their stiffness, sharpening the senses, increasing self-esteem and sociability are some of the ways of continuing life even with the disease. When you start a physical activity, whether it's done actively or passively, your body responds positively. This is why dance, yoga, sports and exercise are important. Massage, physiotherapy, acupuncture, music therapy, hypnosis, spirituality, art and proper nutrition are important allies that can contribute to improving the quality of life of people with Parkinson's disease (quoted in PARKINSON, 2016).

3.3 MASSAGE

The practice of rubbing the body is as instinctive and ancient as man himself because touching oneself or another person is a natural human act. When someone hurts themselves, they automatically try to relieve the pain by massaging the area. As the act of rubbing or massaging promotes greater circulation, oxygenation and local heating, the result will be pain relief (BRAUN; SIMONSON, 2007).

The origins of massage date back to prehistoric times and there are reports, according to historians, that it was already practised in the Ancient Ages by the Persians, Egyptians, Indians and Japanese. According to archaeological studies, prehistoric man already used body friction as a way of relieving pain and injuries. Records from ancient civilisations refer to the benefits of massage around 300 BC (BRAUN; SIMONSON, 2007).

The first to recognise the benefits of the technique of rubbing the body were the Chinese 2,500 BC, recorded in the medical text Huiandgi Nei-Ching, the book of the Yellow Emperor with the amma or amna style (PEREZ; OLIVEIRA, 2015). 1,000 BC Japanese monks studied Buddhism in China and took their knowledge back to Japan. There, new combinations were added (BRAUN; SIMONSON, 2007).

In India, around 1,700 BC, Ayurvedic medicine was practised with massages and herbal treatments. Cherokee and Navajo natives in America used the practice of warming and massaging with herbs to reduce various pains and colic in children. Egyptians, Indians, Persians and Japanese used massage to treat various illnesses and until around the fifth century AD, it was part of the medical treatment of the time (LACROIX, 2014).

According to Perez and Oliveira (2015), the term massage has several origins. In Greek *masso* or *massein* (to squeeze, knead), in Arabic *mass (to massage), in* French *masser* or *massage (to* squeeze, rub, beat), in Latin *fríctio* (friction). The term *therapeutikós,* also of Greek origin, refers to the performance of a medical treatment. The father of medicine Hippocrates (460 to 377 BC) and Claudius Galen (130 to 201 AD) also considered the importance of friction on muscle fibres to regain strength, moderate fatigue and muscle pain.

The history of massage is long and dates back many centuries. The practice has been given different names in various countries and in all of them it has proved to be an effective way of combating pain, maintaining health and recovering from illness. It contributes to the physical, mental and spiritual well-being of individuals, since by working on the whole, it makes the person stronger, safer and more aware (BRAUN; SIMONSON, 2007).

There are many types of massage available today, such as lymphatic drainage, tuina, shiatsu, zen shiatsu, reflexology, ayurveda, classical or therapeutic, among others. Depending on the expected end goal or the patient's clinical condition, one technique or another is best suited to the case. However, they all have in common the improvement and general well-being of the patient, the reduction of pain and the search for the individual's physical, psychological, emotional and energetic balance (BRAUN; SIMONSON, 2007).

3.4 MASSAGE THERAPY AND PAIN

Massage therapy, also known as classical, relaxing or Swedish massage, consists of manipulating the soft tissues of the body and can be defined as methodical, rhythmic compression with the aim of relaxing the muscles and blood flow (CASSAR, 2001).

Its main focus is the relaxation of muscle fibres, which is why it was chosen to be applied in this study, primarily to reduce tremors, stiffness and tension observed in patients with Parkinson's disease.

According to some dictionaries, pain is a sensation of suffering resulting from injury and perceived by specialised nerve formations.

It is perceived differently by people and can appear in cases of insomnia, sadness or fear, as well as being present in anxious and depressed people. It can be minor or major or disappear when we are well, happy, carefree, sleeping well, hopeful or in a pleasant environment. It can be acute, when it results from muscle strain, infections, falls or minor burns, or it can be chronic: serious injuries, spinal problems, amputations, sections of nerves or ageing (PAIN TREATMENT, 2006).

Painful impulses are conducted through the Central Nervous System along the spinal and cranial nerves to the thalamus, where they are transmitted to the parietal lobe in the cerebral cortex, where pain actually occurs and is felt. It is in the cerebral cortex that awareness of the painful process and the type and intensity of pain are processed (MENSE; SIMONS; RUSSEL, 2008). According to the authors, there are areas in the brain that, when activated, release opiate substances such as endorphins, dynorphins, enkephalins, serotonin, noradrenalin and others. These are substances that modulate pain, as they act as inhibitory neurotransmitters. The Behavioural Theory (proposed in 1965 by scientists Melzack and Wall) is based on how certain mechanisms can reduce or suppress the perception of pain by stimulating inhibitory interneurons. It establishes the idea that a non-painful stimulus, in this case massage, can block or modulate the transmission of a harmful stimulus to the Central Nervous System (TREATMENT OF PAIN, 2006).

When the tactile pathway is activated (by the touch of the massage) the pain pathway is inhibited/modulated, so the Pain Gate is partially closed for the transmission of pain and becomes open for the transmission of touch, sensory information (MENSE; SIMONS; RUSSEL, 2008).

Although massage therapy is carried out on the skin, it has effects on all the body's systems, including the central nervous system as a reflex effect. These effects refer to the release of feel-good substances such as endorphins and serotonins and the modulation of pain through the stimulus of touch, relieving anxiety and tension (TREATMENT OF PAIN, 2006).

Other positive effects are mechanical and physiological. According to Teixeira (2006), the mechanical effects of compression, traction, cooling, pressure and friction promote increased joint mobility, stimulation of visceral functions, mobilisation of the treated tissues, local hyperemia, drainage of venous blood and lymph.

The inhibitory neuromuscular effects act on immediate well-being, pain relief and local and general muscle relaxation. In turn, the excitatory neuromuscular effects promote an increase in heart rate and reflex tone, stimulation of the sweat glands and peristaltic movement (TREATMENT OF PAIN, 2006).

Cassar (2001) reports that the therapeutic value of massage extends beyond relaxation. Most massage movements have the additional therapeutic effects of relieving muscle tension and improving circulation. In this way, massage is applied not to cure a disorder, but mainly to treat certain symptoms.

There are countless benefits to massage, not only because of the relaxing effect it has on the physical body, but it is also beneficial for various problems with emotional causes, as the touch conveys support, affection, comfort and acceptance. Throughout the massage process, the hands touch the patient, transmitting trust and helping to reduce anxiety. When the traumas of a person's life have not been overcome, they can become, over time, stiffened muscles and fasciae, resulting in tension and pain that will compromise quality of life (DONATELLI, 2015).

Seubert (2008) reports that the purpose of massage is to make the individual more aware of their own body, as it allows them to get to know their tensions, their breathing and the reflexes that emotional causes provoke in the organism. As a therapeutic resource, it has been recognised as one of the most effective therapies for relieving pain and pain caused by genetic, traumatic or neurological diseases, which generate emotional alterations since the psyche is not separate from the body.

Cassar (2001) reports that relaxation is essential to combat many psychological and emotional states, and massage is one of the best methods for this. Gliding and other manoeuvres can be performed in a calm manner, leading to a reduction in tension. Gentle kneading induces tranquillity, as does scalp massage.

According *to* the author, hand and foot massage and mobilisation movements are effective and result in relaxation. Massage relieves muscle tension and helps to normalise rigid posture patterns, for example when a patient has muscle tension due to anxiety. Respiratory rate can be restored and insomnia, caused by stress, can also be alleviated, since relaxing massage promotes sleep through its movements. "[...] massage brings the person to a point where the mind can heal" (CASSAR, 2001).

Seubert (2008) also emphasises that therapeutic massage, by providing greater contact with the patient's skin (therapeutic touch), generates a greater feeling of welcome, well-being and trust, as well as expanding body awareness, improving perception and sensitivity.

The experience of therapeutic touch induces the individual to get in touch with themselves, to turn inwards, which for many brings peace of mind. For most people, being touched is a pleasant sensation. Through massage, the therapist leads the person to broaden their perception of the regions of their body, sharpening their concentration and providing relaxation (BRAUNSTEIN *et al,* 2011).

It is therefore understood that massage therapy, with its slow, light and rhythmic movements, has beneficial effects on the whole body, as it relaxes the muscles and consequently relieves pain, reduces nervous tension, calms and lowers stress levels (ABREU *et al,* 2012).

3.5 MASSAGE THERAPY AND PARKINSON'S DISEASE

In people with Parkinson's disease, muscle tension is a characteristic feature, which affects the nerves and causes pain. For this reason, it is believed that when they undergo a massage session, muscle tension will be reduced, leading the muscles to stop contracting, through better blood irrigation, a greater flow of nutrients and oxygenation to all tissues and organs. A body with more relaxed muscles will help with emotional and psychological maintenance, reducing anxiety, anguish and insomnia (SEUBERT; VERONESE, 2008).

Abdominal massage can also be very effective against intestinal disorders. Its medicinal use, however, is quite delicate, and it can only be carried out when there is a precise diagnosis and when the therapist knows exactly the results they should achieve (BRAGA *et al,* 2013).

Although doctors still don't usually recommend massage to people with Parkinson's disease as a complementary or alternative treatment, "massage therapy has been shown to be an effective alternative for the treatment of constipation" (BRAZ *etal,* 2013, p.42).

The author says:

> [...] among the various treatment modalities for intestinal constipation (IC), therapeutic massage, especially abdominal massage, is considered to be of great value because, when properly used, it is a simple, non-invasive, effective, low-cost procedure, without many contraindications and without major deleterious effects. This procedure acts on the parasympathetic nervous system, which is responsible for stimulating the motility of the gastrointestinal tract, speeding up the transit of faeces.

Werner (2005, p. 178) reports that:

> Patients with Parkinson's disease experience progressive inflexibility and rigidity of the voluntary muscles. Massage, administered by a therapist who is part of a healthcare team,

can be a valuable tool not only for maintaining flexibility and range of movement, but also for reducing anxiety and depression.

For these reasons, the aim of this study was to add to other scientific studies already published and to confirm that massage can help people with Parkinson's Disease to alleviate the symptoms of the disease.

CHAPTER 4

4 METHODOLOGICAL PROCEDURES

This study was developed and applied by three students on the Massage Therapy Technician course at the Federal Institute of Paraná - Londrina Campus, with the aim of presenting the final data as their final course work, under the guidance of the course lecturers.

The aim was to find out whether massage therapy improves the symptoms of people with Parkinson's disease and, to this end, an exploratory approach was applied to the research.

4.1 POPULATION AND SAMPLE

The participants in the project were located by posting them on the social network page of the Federal Institute of Paraná - Londrina Campus, by the professional responsible for the publications on the network and with the prior authorisation of the coordination of the Technical Course in Massage Therapy. For this purpose, digital artwork was created which included the title of the research, the number of sessions, the duration of each session, the times of the sessions, the students' contact details and the campus address.

It was also publicised on the social networks of the therapists in charge, as well as verbally to people in their social circle. Course lecturers, classmates, friends and acquaintances who expressed sympathy for the topic also helped spread the word about the project.

For inclusion and participation in the study, it was essential that the participants had been diagnosed with Parkinson's Disease by a specialist doctor. It was also necessary that they were not taking part in any other project or programme aimed at Parkinson's sufferers in any institution and that they maintained the intake of medication prescribed by their doctors, as well as the normality of their daily activities. They were asked to avoid missing their weekly appointments as much as possible so that their continuity would not be interrupted. Gender, age or length of time with the condition were not used as exclusion factors.

4.2 DATA COLLECTION METHOD

The first contacts were made by telephone, at which point the face-to-face interviews were scheduled. The interviews confirmed the diagnoses, the interest in taking part in the project and the other criteria needed to take part in the consultations. They were also given all the information about the project, as well as its objectives and procedures, and any doubts were answered. All the participants filled in the Informed Consent Form (APPENDIX 1) and then answered an Assessment Form with 60 questions about Parkinson's Disease (APPENDIX 2), as well as its signs and symptoms. All those responsible for the project were present at all the interviews.

The sessions were held in the Massage Therapy I laboratory at the Federal Institute of Paraná - Londrina Campus, in the afternoon. The space was specially selected because it was located on the ground floor and had toilets and drinking fountains nearby, making it easy for patients to move around if necessary. It also had air conditioning (hot/cold) and a stereo. Three portable stretchers were set up in parallel, enabling the three researchers to attend to patients at the same time. The cream used in the procedure was the same for all the sessions and for all the project participants.

The interventions took place on a weekly basis, with massage therapy sessions lasting one hour and ten minutes. Manoeuvres from the respective technique, an evolution questionnaire and interviews related to the progression of the treatment were used to obtain data.

Patients were assigned to each of the students by random draw, as follows: patients A and B to the first, patients C and F to the second and patients D and E to the third. During the ten massage sessions, there were no changes of patients between the researchers. This criterion was established in order to maintain the bond of trust that exists between patient and therapist, which contributes to the smooth development of the work.

Throughout the research, the same care routine was carried out, which included reaching all body extensions, applied in ventral and dorsal decubitus, bilaterally, involving the sequence of manoeuvres shown in APPENDIX 5.

The elements of the Evaluation Form and Conclusion Form were tabulated in order to organise and facilitate analytical access to the patients' personal data and their findings before treatment began.

The evolution sheets were analysed qualitatively by observing the information recorded by the patients, as well as the notes made by the therapists about each specific treatment.

The final interviews were all transcribed to make it possible to collect as much information as possible that wasn't on any of the other forms/questionnaires applied during treatment.

Through these tools applied in the assessment of patients, the information collected was presented in a descriptive manner with reports and statements from the participants themselves, as well as analysing and discussing the main symptoms observed in the Parkinson's patients treated by this project.

4.3 COLLECTION INSTRUMENTS

The Assessment Form contained the participant's personal information and contact details. It included questions about the length of time they had been suffering from the condition, the medication they were taking, whether they were taking any alternative treatments, whether they had ever been diagnosed with Parkinson's Disease in the family, whether they had any other condition and were undergoing treatment for it, whether they were involved in physical activity (which activity, frequency and duration, and whether it had been recommended by a doctor). Questions were also asked about the practice of massage (whether they had ever received any type of massage and what their expectations were in relation to treatment with the therapy), as well as questions directly related to the symptoms of the disease: sleep disorders, muscle stiffness, tremors, depression, constipation, tiredness, non-specific pain, speech difficulties and swallowing difficulties.

The Progress Form, applied before the start of each appointment, had a visual scale for the patient to mark the level of the symptoms mentioned above, made up with images to make marking easier and more didactic (considering the possibility of them having some intellectual difficulty). There was also a field containing a drawing of the human body (from the front and back) so that the location of possible areas of pain and discomfort could be marked, and another space available so that the patient could describe and say how their days had gone in the last week, from the last appointment to the current one. Included in this document was an exclusive area for the students to indicate whether there had been a reduction in pain and tremors and whether the patient had been able to relax or sleep during the session, plus a field for them to transcribe details of the respective treatment.

At the end of the ten massage sessions, each of the participants filled in the Completion Form and was interviewed individually by two students. They were asked about the project, what they had noticed in their daily lives during the time they had taken part, both physically and emotionally. They were also asked about the relevance or otherwise of the project, whether they would recommend the massage to someone with Parkinson's disease and why, and whether they would continue with the massage if they were able to.

CHAPTER 5

5 ANALYSING AND DISCUSSING THE RESULTS

The patients were named and organised in alphabetical order, of which we have listed some information. All of them, according to the pre-established criteria for exclusion/inclusion in the project, were taking medication for Parkinson's Disease (Prolopa, Entacapone, Azilect), prescribed by their doctors.

Patient A:

Born in April 1958

Married, with children, no paid work;

Diagnosed with Parkinson's disease six years ago.

Patient B:

Born in March 1941

Married, with children, no paid work;

Diagnosed with Parkinson's disease eight years ago.

Patient C:

Born in June 1946

Married, with children, retired;

Diagnosed with Parkinson's disease two years ago.

Patient D:

Born in November 1956

Separated, with children, retired;

Diagnosed with Parkinson's disease three years ago.

Patient E:

Born in August 1951

Married, with children, retired;

Diagnosed with Parkinson's disease three years ago.

Patient F:

Born in March 1964

Married, *with* children, retired;

Diagnosed with Parkinson's disease a year ago.

The ages of the six patients ranged from 53 to 76, four of them men and two women. Among them, the time since they were diagnosed with Parkinson's Disease ranged from one to eight years, respectively.

TABLE 1 Age of participants and time since diagnosis.

	Patient A	Patient B	Patient C	Patient D	Patient E	Patient F
Age	59	76	71	61	66	53
Time to diagnosis of pathology	6	8	2	3	3	1

TABLE 1 Symptoms reported by patients on the Evaluation Form.

		Patient A	Patient B	Patient C	Patient D	Patient E	Patient F
SYMPTOMS	*Sleep disorders*				X	X	X
	Muscle stiffness	X	X	X	X	X	X
	Tremors	X	X	X	X	X	X
	Depression		X				X
	Constipation	X	X				X
	Tiredness		X	X	X		X
	Non-specific pain	X	X				
	Difficulty speaking	X	X		X		X
	Difficulty swallowing						
	Others						

Based on the data shown in Table 1, it can be seen that some symptoms were not reported by any of the participants on the Assessment Sheets. However, as soon as the sessions began, important additional information was collected from the progress sheets filled in before each session about the different symptoms reported by the patients themselves, which became the object of analysis in this research because they were mentioned by a greater number of participants throughout the sessions than the symptoms previously reported on the assessment sheet, and refer to: sleep disorders, anxiety, non-specific pain, tremor and stiffness and constipation (TABLE 2).

TABLE 2 Symptoms reported by patients during appointments.

		Patient A	Patient B	Patient C	Patient D	Patient E	Patient F
SYMPTOMS	*Sleep disorders*		X		X	X	X
	Muscle stiffness	X	X	X	X	X	X
	Tremors	X	X	X	X	X	X
	Constipation	X	X				X
	Tiredness		X	X	X		
	Non-specific pain	X	X	X	X		X
	Speech difficulties				X		
	Anxiety	X	X	X	X	X	X

5.   1SLEEP DISORDERS

The data obtained in the study showed that it was favourable to improve the quality of sleep in people with Parkinson's disease after receiving massage therapy sessions. In the sessions given to six patients during the research, we obtained important responses in relation to the sleep symptom.

Patient D reported that when he is anxious, he loses sleep or wakes up very early, outside of normal hours, and so with the practice of massage he noticed a significant improvement, especially in the two days following the massage.

Patient E reported on his second visit: "On the day of the massage, I went to sleep as soon as I got home". In the interview at the end of the project, when asked if he had noticed any improvement in his sleep, he commented: "So I improve a lot after the massage. My quality of sleep improves on the day of the massage".

Patient F, in his fourth consultation, reported that: "due to the tremors which have been intense over the last few days, I have not been able to sleep for the last week", thus a direct relationship between insomnia and the tremors was observed.

Sleeping is a common activity and need for most animals. In humans, sleep needs vary from 4 to 10 hours every 24 hours.

> **The quality and quantity of sleep should be assessed by bedtime, sleep latency (time from bedtime to falling asleep), number and time of awakenings, final morning rising and waking time, and frequency and duration of naps (BEERS, 2008, p. 2021).**

The author states that there are two types of sleep: NREM, without rapid eye movements, and REM with rapid eye movements, and in both there are physiological changes, so sleep cannot be seen as a passive, monotonous activity (BEERS, 2008).

Sleep occurs in five distinct phases or stages where, in stage I, sleep is light and the person can be woken up easily. In stage II, the eyes stop moving. In stage III, brain waves are slower. In stage IV, only delta waves are emitted by the brain (responsible for deep sleep) and the body also secretes hormones that develop growth in children and adolescents and repair and regeneration in adults. In the REM (Rapid Eye Movement) stage, dreams occur, the eyes move quickly and muscle activity in the limbs is usually absent (WERNER, 2005).

Stages III and IV are known as deep sleep and are where people spend the longest at the beginning of the night. REM sleep occurs in the morning and stage I is where the person spends the most time. It takes 90 to 100 minutes to complete a sleep cycle, after which the whole cycle restarts again (WERNER, 2005).

The stages of sleep are cyclical and each one fulfils a specific function designed to keep the body healthy. It is a necessary and vital process for health and without balanced sleep, we can develop disorders that seriously compromise our health, such as slow reflexes, reduced cognitive abilities, impairment of the immune system: chronic pain, depression, hallucinations and psychosis, fibromyalgia syndrome (WERNER, 2005).

Beers (2008, p.2026) states that "physical disorders can interfere with sleep, and disorders that cause pain or discomfort, particularly those that worsen with movement, cause transient awakenings and poor sleep quality". For Borges, *et al* (2010) sleep disorders are treatable and, if not, can have a significant adverse effect on the quality of life of these patients.

> Patients with Parkinson's disease experience a wide range of sleep disorders, from a complete reversal of normal sleep patterns to insomnia, as it is difficult or impossible for them to move around in bed (WERNER, 2005, p.177).

According to Borges, *et al* (2010) sleep disorders are frequent in patients with Parkinson's disease, with between 60% and 83% of patients suffering from insomnia. Various factors contribute to impairing the patient's sleep, among which the most common are tremors, which can become more frequent at night.

Even when they manage to fall asleep, the patient ends up waking up several times, which prevents them from reaching the deeper stages of sleep. Without restorative sleep, the risk of daytime sleepiness is even greater

According to the same author, another factor that can aggravate insomnia symptoms is depression or emotional and psychological factors, which are common problems in people with the disease. Insomnia in Parkinson's disease has a multifactorial origin related to age, the pathological process or secondary to factors associated with PD such as painful dystonia, cramps, re-emergence of nocturnal parkinsonism symptoms, mood disorders, psychosis, sleep apnoea, nocturia, poor sleep hygiene, motor disorders (restless legs syndrome, periodic movement of extremities, REM sleep behaviour disorder) and the effect of drugs used to treat motor symptoms.

There are more than 70 sleep-related disorders that make it difficult to get enough sleep or wake up refreshed, and according to Werner (2005), older people feel less refreshed by sleep because these disorders increase with age. For the author, massage is indicated for people who are affected by such disorders, as it can improve the quality of sleep and reduce mental and physical stresses that can interfere with sleep, as well as increasing the time of stages III or IV, which are restorative stages that reduce the sensation of pain and speed up healing.

> Massage is certainly indicated for most types of sleep disorders. Some studies indicate that massage increases the amount of time spent in Stage III or IV restorative sleep, which reduces the sensation of pain (WERNER, 2005, p.250).

As it is a chronic and progressive condition, regular massage therapy is essential in the life of a person with Parkinson's Disease (VERSAGI, 2015). For the author, anxiety, fears, the very physical restlessness characteristic of the disease, as well as the inability to change position in bed, lead to insomnia. This is why massage is important for people with Parkinson's disease. And when they experience depression, anxiety, restlessness and insomnia, massage can reduce these symptoms with relaxation techniques that take the patient into a relaxed, parasympathetic state, i.e. calm.

5.2 ANXIETY

All the patients seen during the study reported an improvement in their emotional well-being. These patients did not have reports of psychological disorders, but during the assessment and consultations they provided important information about their emotional states, even though this symptom was not listed as an option on the Assessment Form (APPENDIX 2). In this way, massage proved to be beneficial and effective, as we can see from the patients' statements.

Patient A said in the interview that there had been changes in her emotions during the time she had received the massage and that it was her family who had noticed this change: "People at home have commented that I'm calmer now. My son who lives abroad said I'm more relaxed and calm. Before I was more nervous, more tense.

Patient B also spoke about the changes in her emotions: "I used to be more nervous, I wanted more, to receive more (attention from everyone), now I don't". Patient C said in the final interview that "the massage gave you more energy, you start to relax more, you become calmer".

What was reported by the respective patients is in line with Cassar's (2001) report that massage can help people with Parkinson's disease as it is indicated for those who are going through a complex health situation and are also emotionally sensitive, in the case of depression and anxiety. Through the physical contact that massage provides, sufferers feel accepted and cared for, which increases their self-esteem.

Patient D said that "the massage only improved my anxiety. The massage helped me a lot because it released some hormones and I'm more energised, more willing, less anxious". On the eighth session, he wrote on his evaluation form that the anxiety, as well as the tremors and stiffness, improved in the first three days of the massage, but that from the fourth day onwards, he felt anxious again because the physical symptoms in his body began to return.

According to Bonnet (2009), generalised anxiety disorder is characterised by excessive preoccupation with the problems of everyday life (which is difficult to control) and generates problems related to concentration, agitation, internal tension, fatigability, acts of failure, irritation, sleep disturbances and tense muscles. It is the most frequent psychological problem in the general population, after depression, and tends to become more pronounced with the onset of Parkinson's Disease, as it is a frequent symptom in sufferers, since the pathology itself tends to generate feelings of restlessness, either because of the physical limitations they are subjected to or because of the emotional apprehensions they tend to face. In addition to these factors, dopaminergic treatments and the progression of the disease can contribute to anxiety in general.

Massage is recommended for people with Parkinson's disease, since relaxation techniques, breathing exercises and body therapies are considered excellent resources for patients with anxiety, so the results of this study show that massage therapy is an appropriate choice for patients with this disease.

During the project, we were able to observe the anxiety reported and demonstrated by the patients at the beginning of the sessions and the tranquillity they showed at the end of the service.

Patient E reported:

"Massage brings about changes, my family has noticed, they say I'm calmer, calmer. Massage improves people's self-esteem a lot [...] I don't understand why massage isn't recommended by doctors when it gives very good results, because I'm noticing improvements in my body, in

From the third session onwards, patient F reported that he felt more relaxed and calm and less anxious at the end of the massage, unlike when he arrived. At the last appointment, in his interview, he reported the benefits he had seen because he felt calmer and better about his anxiety.

> "When you're nervous, remembering the tranquillity of the massage, the peace you feel, helps you make better decisions. You become calmer, you learn to be calm. With massage, the body relaxes. Massage brings more peace and tranquillity and it's not just the body, it's the mind too."

For Werner (2005), massage is not only beneficial for reducing the rigidity and inflexibility that are progressive in Parkinson's Disease, but it is also important for reducing anxiety and depression.

> Massage also promotes a deeper, more natural breathing pattern. Doing so regularly relaxes muscles, nerves, bones and the whole body. It aids the digestive system, maintaining balance and the correct circulation of body gases; it induces deep sleep, increases appetite, and generally makes life more joyful (JOHARI, 1996, p.18).

With the stimulation provided by massage manoeuvres, the body calms down and relaxes, the muscles become more flexible, the mind quiets down and the nervous system functions in a balanced way. Massage helps the mind to become calmer and less agitated (CARDIM, 2012).

5.3 NON-SPECIFIC PAIN

Among the patients seen during the study, three had pain classified as non-specific, according to Chart 2. Pain affects many people with Parkinson's disease, reducing their quality of life. Different types of pain have been described, but their related pathophysiological mechanisms are still unclear (GANDOLFI *etal,* 2017).

Pain in people with Parkinson's disease is not always related to the symptoms of muscle rigidity, dystonia or other motor disability. The pain is related to the disease itself and reported as vague and diffuse. They can be described as burning, tingling, numbing pains that cause a lot of discomfort. They also don't improve with painkillers or anti-inflammatories (LETRO, 2007).

Patient C had pain in the hip and ankle regions during the study, but during the course of the treatment he reported improvement, saying that after the fifth massage session he no longer felt pain in the ankle region and was able to walk normally. After the eighth session, he said he no longer felt pain in the hip area, as confirmed by his report: "The pain went away first, right, it decreased more, and I don't know, the strength seems to have increased as well, the tiredness, all that. The pain went away. God forbid, if I had the pain I'd ask to die many times".

Pain, according to Pimenta and Silva (2008, p.645) is an unpleasant emotional and sensory experience and "one of the most frequent reasons for disability and suffering for patients with a serious illness in progression".

Patient D reported an improvement in his pain after the second, third and eighth sessions, and in the last interview of the project he concluded: "Certain points of my body hurt and I noticed that now it doesn't anymore, the pain in my leg, in my lower back. Suddenly it all went away and I felt really good, I'm fine".

In a study carried out in Germany with 178 people with Parkinson's disease, all reported pain as the most distressing symptom, which most impairs their ability to carry out daily activities and which is not always relieved by anti-Parkinsonian drugs. Pain is frequent, complex, impairs quality of life and is associated with depression and anxiety. It can also occur due to the disease itself (BUHMANN, *etal.*, 2017).

For this reason, it can be extremely difficult for patients with advanced illnesses to find a language to describe their pain, not only because it is an experience that bears no resemblance to any previous sensation, but also because of its emotional, social and spiritual components (PIMENTA; SILVA, 2008).

Patient F complained of lower back and shoulder pain and noted the benefits of massage for pain relief and general well-being:

> *"You start to relax and it goes away. Because I was in a lot of pain even before. It was terrible, it bothered me, you couldn't talk to anyone because you were in so much pain. And every time I was in pain I got nervous, it hurt even more. I used to take 3, 4, 5 tablets to get rid of the pain. Today I don't do that any more. I began to realise that this business (massage) doesn't just affect the physical, just the muscles, just the pain in the body. It goes to the mind as well. The way you talk, the way you behave, everything starts to change.*

Many factors influence pain symptoms, including "fatigue, depression, anger, fear, anxiety about the disease and feelings of hopelessness and helplessness" (PIMENTA; SILVA, 2008, p. 646). The authors also emphasise that the effectiveness of pain relief will depend on the cause of the symptom and that intervention measures can vary between the use of drugs or non-pharmacological treatments, including massage therapy, as it "acts to improve circulation, promoting muscle relaxation and relieving psychological tension" (IBID., p. 651).

> Emotional factors such as expectation, anxiety and fear can influence the perception of pain. The greater the tension in the individual, the stronger their perception of pain; conversely, the more relaxed the subject, the less intense the pain seems to be. [...] relaxation, such as that obtained through massage, can be fundamental in reducing pain. (CASSAR, 2001, p.40)

Another reference to the use of massage therapy as an ally in the treatment of non-specific pain is made by Chiba and Ashmawi (2016) when they refer to the various techniques that can be used (shiatsu, do-in, reflex zone, among others), depending on the problem presented.

According to Field (2014), massage with moderate pressure has positive effects, including reducing pain in different syndromes, reducing depression and anxiety

Kneading, sliding, rubbing and tapping manoeuvres help to activate the nervous, circulatory and lymphatic systems, promoting physical and mental relaxation. In therapeutic massage, the use of gentle, continuous movements performed with the hands stimulates the production of hormones responsible for relaxation (endorphins, serotonin, oxytocin), thus reducing anxiety, relieving tension and pain (VERSAGI, 2015).

Massage as an alternative treatment does not provide a cure for the disease, but it does promote relief and well-being since it acts to control psychological, emotional and physical symptoms such as depression, anxiety and pain. By promoting relaxation and well-being, massage contributes to a better quality of life (CAÍRES, *et al,* 2014).

5.4 MUSCLE RIGIDITY AND TREMOR

Parkinson's disease is a neurodegenerative disease characterised by motor symptoms such as: rigidity, bradykinesia, rest tremor and postural instability and non-motor symptoms such as: neuropsychiatric, sleep, autonomic and sensory disorders (BORGES, *etal,* 2010).

The main symptoms presented by the patients during the study were related to motor aspects, especially tremor and rigidity (as shown in Chart 2). These symptoms were reported by the patients at the initial assessment and were observed throughout the appointments.

According to Cassar (2001), the three main signs that characterise Parkinson's Disease (which become evident as the disease progresses) are muscle rigidity or muscle spasm, resting tremor and bradykinesia (abnormal slowness of voluntary movements).

The benefits of massage therapy were proven by the patients' statements in the final interview, as well as in reports during the appointments.

Stiffness is an involuntary "increase in muscle tone, triggered during passive movement of the limbs, neck or trunk through the full range of motion. It affects the whole body and is most evident in the extremities." (BARROS *et al,* 2006, p. 24). It is generally limited to the muscles of a particular action, affecting both agonist and antagonist muscles (BONNET; HERGUETA, 2009).

Muscle rigidity is a symptom that greatly compromises the quality of life of people with Parkinson's disease.

> Patients with Parkinson's disease experience progressive inflexibility and rigidity of the voluntary muscles. Massage can be a valuable tool not only for maintaining flexibility and range of movement, but also for reducing anxiety and depression. (WERNER, 2005, p.177)

Patient E, who had stiffness in his right upper limb and right lower limb, asked in the second session for the manoeuvres to be "stronger" in these places as he felt better, and in the seventh session he wrote on his evaluation form that "the *massages are great, they help with stiffness and tremors".*

Patient F reported in his interview significant improvements in aspects related to stiffness after starting treatment with massage therapy:

> *"That stiffness, that thing that gives, that nervousness that feels like it's going to burst your nerves, right? You can control it, you can remember how the massage was done, that moment. Even though you don't say anything, the movements, the sensation start to dominate you. You start to relax. You're in control of relaxing.*

Patient C, on the other hand, reported improved walking during the interview:

> *"I've improved a lot when it comes to walking too, I'm walking every day. It's given us more energy and pep, so this (massage) has been very good. It seems that we've even developed to walk, I walk faster than before. It was the massage, I have no doubt. Before, I walked more slowly, I couldn't walk much. Before I couldn't do it, I'd walk from here to the house, I'd arrive tired, so it's improved. That's why I say, I recommend it to anyone, do it (massage) because it's good".*

In people with Parkinson's disease, stiffness is observed in a resting position or when the joints are passively mobilised and can be intensified when performing an atypical movement, in states of mental concentration or emotional tension. It can be continuous, also called "lead pipe" or intermittent with episodes of sudden muscle relaxation ("cogwheel"). It is usually reported as muscle tension and contributes to motor difficulty, which is the main characteristic of the illness (BONNET; HERGUETA, 2009, p. 22).

According to Barras, *et al* (2006), as well as limiting movement in all its amplitude (hypokinesia), muscle rigidity directly interferes with the balance of Parkinson's disease patients by simultaneously increasing the tone of the agonist and antagonist muscles, hindering communication between the muscles' praprioceptive receptors and the capacity for postural muscle activity. This leads to difficulties in rotating the trunk and head, which are fundamental for adjusting the individual's posture and balance, as stated by patient D during the interview:

> *"I used to lose my balance when I walked and my legs would get too tired, even when I was doing physical exercises. I feel like I can stand up for longer, I can also leave my house and go to the centre on foot."*

When performing a movement, for every muscle group that performs it (agonists), there is another muscle group with opposing activities (antagonists). When muscles are activated to perform a certain activity, others are inhibited in order to facilitate the same movement. In Parkinson's disease, this inhibition is not carried out effectively because some commands originating in the cerebral cortex reach the muscles in an altered way due to the pathology (BARROS *et al*, 2006).

> Massage is indicated to relieve muscle tension and maintain joint mobility. Treatment can be applied in the early stages and continued as the condition progresses, as long as it doesn't cause any discomfort. Sliding manoeuvres are therefore beneficial for systemic circulation and for circulation in stiff muscles. Techniques such as compression and kneading further reduce muscle tension and passively stretch the tissues (CASSAR, 2001, p.74).

One of the most striking symptoms of Parkinson's disease is the presence of tremors. Of the research participants, five had this symptom, which was identified during the assessment, noted during the consultations and at the end of the interview process.

Patient B, in his first sessions, had shoulder tremors that persisted throughout the massage and stretches. The intensity of the tremors fluctuated over the course of the sessions, showing that emotional aspects experienced at the time directly influenced the occurrence of this symptom. At the end of the ten sessions, the patient had very mild tremors.

The term tremor is defined by Campbell (2009) as a movement that occurs involuntarily and is characterised by rhythmic oscillations (shaking or shuddering) of a part of the body. They are divided into two groups: rest tremor or passive tremor and movement tremor. Parkinsonism is related to resting tremor. Beers (2008) says that resting tremors are maximal at rest and decrease with activity; it is usually one of the symptoms of Parkinson's disease.

Patient C presented the symptom of tremor to a lesser degree during the treatment, but over the course of the sessions he reported a good mood for walking and a significant reduction in this symptom. In the last sessions, tremor was not observed. When the patient was asked in the final interview about the benefits he felt from the massage, he reported: *"[...] the massage reduced the trembling I had"*, *"[...] now that it's cold, we feel it more, because we want to hold in the cold, right, (laughs), so it seems that the muscles aren't relaxed, right"*.

With patient D it was possible to have a good observation and proof of the acute effect of massage therapy for Parkinson's Disease. The patient reported that in the first three days after the massage he felt very well, without tremors, pain and tingling in his left leg and right hand (reported and observed in the assessment). He also reported a better mood and ability to carry out his activities of daily living. Of particular note here is the patient's statement that on the fourth day after the massage the symptoms returned gradually and increased over the days: *"the first four days I felt very well, after that the tremors started and I felt a bit agonised"*.

The patient said that after the fourth day, he became anxious and that anxiety, as well as personal and emotional problems, accentuated the symptoms. In the seventh session, the patient reported that he could feel the soles of his feet again when stepping and walking, and that this sensitivity had previously been compromised. Another observation made by the patient was the improvement in his voice, which according to him failed at different times. At the end of the treatment, he said in an interview: *"[...now with the massage, the medication has more effect than before. It has a better effect"[...] I felt a satisfactory improvement this week, it was as if I had no problem at all"*.

Patient E's account also shows the benefits of massage therapy: *"Massages are great, they help with stiffness and tremor, they increase self-esteem, especially as it's a continuous syndrome"* and also: *"take care of the body and the soul will follow"*.

Regarding tremors, Ferraz (2011) says that resting tremor is one of the characteristics of Parkinson's disease and can affect any of the four limbs and the chin, as well as the vocal folds. In the hands, it is characterised by the thumb and forefinger touching (rubbing against each other). For him, the tremor tends to diminish or even disappear for a few moments when the affected limb starts moving and the amplitude can be greater or lesser depending on the state of muscle relaxation and emotional stress. This is in line with what was observed in patient D, mentioned above.

Patient F had an intense tremor in his right upper limb. During his first treatment, the noise of his hand hitting the stretcher drew the attention of the therapists and other patients. The tremor persisted with the massage on the other upper limb, but, to the therapist's surprise, when she started the manoeuvres and mobilisations with the right upper limb, the tremor stopped. When he rested the limb on the stretcher to perform manoeuvres on the face, the tremor remained mild compared to the beginning. At the end of this first session, the patient reported relaxation and a reduction in trapezius pain.

In subsequent appointments, it was noted that the patient came to the sessions with a marked tremor and that during the massage of the right upper limb and with the patient's relaxation, this symptom decreased and even disappeared. At the end of the sessions, the patient said in an interview:

> *"Most of the times when my arm stops, when it rests a bit, it's when I get too distracted watching a film. I get too distracted watching a film, then I notice that it stops for a little while,*

According to Borges (2011), tremor is the result of contractions of antagonistic muscles and can be synchronous or alternating. It can be a physiological process, which is present in all people but is not visible, or it can be pathological. It can also be combined in different syndromes. The author also states that parkinsonian tremor can disappear in sleep or during complete relaxation, but that it becomes more intense during walking, in stressful situations and with mental abstractions.

5.5 CONSTIPATION

The term constipation syndrome refers to a set of symptoms and/or signs secondary to various aetiological factors and etiopathogenic mechanisms. Constipation is referred to differently among patients: for some, it is infrequent bowel movements, while for others it represents a great deal of defecation effort, hardened faeces, a feeling of incomplete evacuation and a low number of bowel movements per week (RODRIGUES; ROCHA; ZANANDREA, 2004).

According to Versagi (2015), constipation is more common in women, adults over 65, people who drink too little water and too little dietary fibre, and those who take antidepressants. According to the author, there are two categories of constipation: functional, with easily recognisable causes, and idiopathic, with obscure or unknown causes. The signs or symptoms of constipation are quite obvious and the person usually has: hard, difficult to remove stools, bowel movements less than three times a week, malaise and headaches, gas and a very full abdomen, as well as making a lot of effort in an attempt to evacuate.

Constipation can be a symptom of depression, which reduces the number of bowel movements and the lack of bowel movements increases depression, making the person a chronic user of cathartics, i.e. substances that speed up the defecation process (BEERS, 2008). For the author, in people with Parkinson's disease, constipation is classified as chronic since it is a disorder of the central nervous system, which is also aggravated by the use of anti-Parkinsonian drugs.

Of the patients taking part in the study, three reported a history of constipation (Chart 2).

Patient A, in his second appointment, reported that after the first massage session his bowels worked as soon as he returned home and that he hadn't had a bowel movement for ten days, and that he had bowel movements twice during the week. During the appointments, the patient reported that he had reduced his medication and attributed the improved bowel function to the massage. He told the therapist that he had travelled and forgotten his medication, but still had no difficulty evacuating. In the final interview, the patient reported:

Patient B reported that his bowels worked every day and that he used medication to do so. During the appointments (in the fifth session), the patient reported that he had reduced his medication and was only taking it every other day; in the seventh session, he reported that he was taking a two-day break from medication and yet his bowel movements remained normal.

Patient E, in his third session, reported that his bowels became "looser" after the massages began, which they hadn't been before.

In people with Parkinson's disease, intestinal constipation is very common and appears early. Their bowel habits do not follow a regular pattern, because constipation is an incidence of the disease and its severity is related to the importance of motor problems and the duration of its evolution, leading to discomfort, embarrassment and the continuous use of medication (BONNET, 2009).

The treatment of constipation can follow pharmacological and non-pharmacological measures. Massage techniques can also be used successfully, as they provide rest and relaxation by stimulating the parasympathetic system (VERSAGI, 2015).

Abdominal massage acts on the colon to treat constipation. The application of direct, deep and rhythmic pressure stimulates the body's natural peristaltic action. When the colon is massaged and stimulated, its contents are also worked on.

The manoeuvres on the abdomen should be performed in a clockwise direction, in progressive movements that start superficially but gradually go deeper into the muscles of the abdominal cavity to achieve the desired results. The following are used: kneading, compression, medium and deep pressure, rhythmic movements made with the whole hand or fingertips (VERSAGI, 2015).

The reports made by the patients in this study prove that, according to Domenico and Wood (2008), mechanical stimulation of the abdomen through massage can increase peristalsis, speeding up the emptying of intestinal contents.

In the case of Parkinson's Disease, massage is applied to help relieve some of the symptoms associated with the problem since it is indicated for a pathological condition when it tends to present benefits for treatment (CASSAR, 2001).

CHAPTER 6

6 .FINAL CONSIDERATIONS

During the course of this study, it was observed that massage was effective in all the symptoms analysed: constipation, sleep, reduced anxiety, muscle stiffness, tremor and non-specific pain.

Each patient's improvement was noticed by the team of therapists and also by the patient himself, as well as by family and friends. The six participants achieved results and expressed the gains made in their own way, so it was noted that after starting therapy, daily life became more enjoyable and less dependent as they felt less pain, walked without feeling tired, had fewer tremors, slept better with restorative sleep, bowels worked without the need for daily medication, and were calmer and more peaceful.

Massage proved effective for all the participants, reducing their limitations, embarrassment and dependence. Simple daily actions, which for people with Parkinson's disease represent a great deal, were performed with greater skill after the massage therapy treatment.

This study has shown how comprehensive massage is, providing not only physical effects but also help with drug treatment and improving the quality of life and well-being of patients with Parkinson's disease.

It is undeniable that this is a complex and wide-ranging subject, so it is considered that there is still much to be researched in the area of massage, as well as its health benefits. The authors suggest that further studies be carried out, with a greater number of sessions and participants, involving direct and indirect effects, also proving other benefits. Studies related to the reduction of a specific symptom would also be of great value, increasing the degree of reliability of the data obtained in the present study.

REFERENCES

ABREU, M. F.; SOUZA, T. F.; FAGUNDES, D. S. The effects of massage therapy on physical and psychological stress. **Revista Científica FAEMA,** [S.I.], v. 3, n. 1, p. 101- 105, jun. 2012. Available at: <http://www.faema.edu.br/revistas/index.php/Revista- FAEMA/article/view/119>. Accessed on: 10 May 2017.

BARROS, A. L. S. (Org.) *et al.* **Parkinson's disease:** a multidisciplinary view. São José dos Campos: Pulso, 2006.

BEERS, M. H. (Coord.) **Merck Manual:** diagnosis and treatment. 18 ed. São Paulo: Roca, 2008.

BONNET, A. M.; HERGUETA, T. A **Doença de Parkinson no Dia-a-Dia.** São Paulo: Andrei, 2009.

BORGES, et al. **Parkinson's Disease:** Recommendations. São Paulo: Ominifarma, 2010.

BRAGA, I.R. *et al.* Correlations of isometric shoulder lift strength in the scapular plane and palmar grip with measures of upper limb capacity and performance in individuals with chronic hemiparesis. **Revista Terapia Manual,** São Paulo, v. 10, n. 47, p. 12-18, 2012. Available at: <https://www.submission-mtprehabjournal.com/revista/article/view/59/24>. Accessed on: 10 May

2017.

BRAUN, M. B.; SIMONSON, S. J. **Introduction to massage therapy.** Barueri: Manole, 2007.

BRAUNSTEIN, M. V. G.; BRAZ, M. M.; PIVETTA, H. M. F. **The physiology of massage therapy.** Available at: <http://www.unifra.br/eventos/forumfisio2011/Trabalhos/2246.pdf>. Accessed on: 8 May 2017.

BRAZ, M. M. *et al.* Effects of massage on constipation: a systematic review. **Revista Biomotriz,** Cruz Alta, v. 7, n. 1, jul. 2013, p. 42-52. Available at:

<http://revistaeletronica.unicruz.edu.br/index.php/BIOMOTRIZ/article/view/165/pdf>. Accessed on: 8 May 2017.

BUHMANN, C. *et al.* Pain in Parkinson's disease: a cross-sectional survey of its prevalence, specifics, and therapy. **J. Neurol.,** Berlin, v. 264, n. 4, p. 758-769, apr. 2017. Available at: <https://link-springer-com.ezl O9.periodicos.capes.gov.br/article/10.1007/s00415-017-8426-y>. Accessed on: 17 Oct. 2017.

CAÍRES, Juliana Souza *et al.* The use of complementary therapies in palliative care: benefits and purposes. **Cogitare Enfermagem,** Curitiba, v. 19, n. 3, p. 514-520, Sep. 2014. Available at <http://www.revenf.bvs.br/scielo.php?script=sci_arttext&pid=S1414-   85362014000300012>. Accessed on: 6 Nov. 2017.

CAMBIER, J.; MASSON, M.; DEHEN, H. **Manual de neurologia.** 2. ed. rev. e atual. São Paulo: Masson, 1988.

CARDIM, V. C. **Ayurvedic massage:** science of vitality. 1. ed. Lisbon: Dinalivro, 2012.

CASSAR, M. P. **Manual de massagem terapêutica:** um guia completo de massoterapia para o estudante e para o terapeuta. São Paulo: Manole, 2001.

CHIBA, T., ASHMAWI, H. Diagnosis and treatment of pain. IN: FREITAS, E. V.; PY, L. (Coord.). **treatise on geriatrics and gerontology.** 4. ed. Rio de Janeiro: Guanabara Koogan, 2016.

DONATELLI, S. **The language of touch:** Eastern and Western massage therapy. 1. ed. Rio de Janeiro: Roca, 2015.

DUFOUR, M. *et al.* **Massages and massage therapy:** effects, techniques and applications. São Paulo: Andrei, 2001.

FALCÃO, L. F. R. (Org.). **Manual of neurology.** 1. ed. São Paulo: Roca, 2010.

FERRAZ, H. B. Parkinson's disease In: BERTOLUCCI, P. H. F. *et al.* (Org.). **Guia de neurologia.** Barueri: Manole, 2011. p. 351-372.

FIELD, T. Massage therapy research review. **Complementary Therapies in Clinical Practice,** Amsterdam, v. 20, n. 4, p. 224-229, nov. 2014. Available at: <https://www.ncbi.nlm.nih.gov/pmc/articles/PMC5467308/>. Accessed on: 6 Nov. 2017.

GANDOLFI, M. *et al.* Understanding and treating pain syndromes in parkinson's disease. **International Review of Neurobiology,** New York, v. 134, p. 827-858, 2017. Available at: <http://www.sciencedirect.com/science/article/pii/S0074774217300570via%3Dihub>   . Accessed on: 2 Nov. 2017.

GOMES, J. C. P. Pain in the elderly. IN: TEIXEIRA, M. J.; LIN, T. Y.; KAZIYAMA, H. H. S. (Org.). **Pain:** myofascial pain syndrome and musculoskeletal pain. São Paulo: Roca, 2006.

JOHARI, H. **Ayurvedic massage manual:** traditional Indian techniques for balancing body and mind. São Paulo: Ground, 1996.

LACROIX, N. *et al.* **Complete body massage guide:** illustrated to perfect facial, cephalic, body and reflexology massage techniques. 1. ed. São Paulo: Madras, c2014.

LETRO, G. H. **Pain in Parkinson's disease.** 2007. 79 f. Dissertation (Master's in Medical Sciences) - State University of Campinas, Faculty of Medical Sciences, Campinas, 2007. Available at: <http://repositorio.unicamp.br/bitstream/REPOSIP/309086/1/Letro_GraceHelena_M.p   df>. Accessed on: 2 Nov. 2017.

MARTINS, M. A. (Coord.) *et al.* **Clinical medicine.** Barueri: Manole, 2009.

MENSE, S.; SIMONS, D. G.; RUSSELL, I. J. **Muscle pain:** nature, diagnosis and treatment . 1. ed. Barueri: Manole, 2008.

MOREIRA, C. S. *etal.* Parkinson's disease: how to diagnose and treat it. **Revista Científica da Faculdade de Medicina de Campos,** Campos dos Goytacazes, v. 2, n. 2, p. 19-29, 2007. Available at: <http://www.fmc.br/revista/V2N2P19-29.pdf>. Accessed on: 8 May 2017.

PARKINSON: my special health guide, São Paulo: On Line, 2016.

PEREZ, E.; OLIVEIRA, P. U. **Classic and modern massage therapy techniques.** São Paulo: Érica, 2015.

PIMENTA, F. A. P., SILVA, J. F. Pain control. IN: MORAES, E. N. **Basic principles of geriatrics and gerontology.** Belo Horizonte: COOPMED, 2008.

TEIXEIRA, M. J.; LIN, T. Y.; KAZIYAMA, H. H. S. (Org). Pain: myofascial pain syndrome and musculoskeletal pain . São Paulo: Roca, 2006.

TREATMENT OF PAIN. Rio de Janeiro: Guanabara Koogan, 2006.

TU MA, R. Parkinson's: two centuries. **Carta Capital,** São Paulo, v. 23, n. 959, p. 65, 5 Jul 2017.

VERSAGI, C. M. **Therapeutic massage therapy protocols:** step-by-step techniques for various clinical conditions. 1. ed. Barueri: Manole, 2015.

WERNER, R. **Guia de patologia para massoterapeutas.** 2. ed. Rio de Janeiro: Guanabara Koogan, 2005.

SABINO, L. A. *et al.* The aesthetic benefits of a patient with Parkinson's Disease. **Revista de Iniciação Científica da Universidade Vale do Rio Verde,** Betim, v. 2, n. 2, p. 20, 2012. Available at: <http://periodicos.unincor.br/index.php/iniciacaocientifica/article/view/1761/1425>. Accessed on: 8 May 2017.

SEUBERT, F.; VERONESE, L. Massage therapy assisting in the prevention and treatment of physical and psychological illnesses. In: BRAZILIAN CONGRESS OF CORPORAL PSYCHOTHERAPIES, 8, 2008, Curitiba. **Proceedings...** Curitiba: Reichian Centre, 2008. Available at:

<http://www.centroreichiano.com.br/artigos/Anais%202008/Fabiano%20e%20Liane.p   df>. Accessed on: 8 May 2017.

WOOTEN, G.F. *et al.* Are men at greater risk for Parkinson's disease than women? **Journal of Neurology, Neurosurgery & Psychiatry,** Charlottesville, v. 75, n. 4, p. 637-639, apr. 2004. Available at: <http://jnnp.bmj.eom/content/75/4/637>. Accessed on: 10 May 2017.

APPENDICES

APPENDIX 1: Informed Consent Form

Research title:

"IDENTIFYING THE BENEFITS OF RELAXING MASSAGE ON THE HEALTH AND QUALITY OF

LIFE OF

PATIENTS WITH PARKINSON'S DISEASE"

I, , bearer of ID number[9] and herein referred to as PATIENT, agree to **voluntarily** participate in the respective research which will be carried out at the IFPR - Federal Institute of Paraná located at Rua: João XXIII n[9] 600, city of Londrina/PR. The aim of the research is to find out whether Relaxing Massage can be an effective alternative for improving the quality of life of patients with Parkinson's disease. I am aware that my participation is of great academic importance and will take place through the following activities:

1. *Complete the Patient Assessment Form;*
2. *Answering Qualitative Symptom Questionnaires;*
3. *Receive 10 Relaxing Massage sessions once a week.*

My participation is completely voluntary and gives me the right to refuse to co-operate or to withdraw from the interventions at any time, without any burden or prejudice to either party. I am aware that the information collected will be used entirely and strictly for the purposes of this research and will be treated with complete confidentiality, keeping my identity absolutely confidential.

No PATIENT will pay or be remunerated for participating in this study and all the data and documents involved will be kept completely confidential, under the responsibility of the RESEARCHERS who are developing this study. These materials will be essential for the purposes of their Final Project for the Massage Therapy Technician Course taught at the appropriate educational institution.

In the event of any queries arising after the signing of this document, the RESEARCHERS are at your complete disposal to contact you on the following telephone numbers: 99192-9957 (Anilú), 99617-1303 (Shohreh) and 99943-3435 (Sonia).

We declare that we are aware of the terms established herein and of the research procedures, and so we all sign this agreement in two copies of equal content.

Londrina, 2017.

Researchers in charge:

Anilú Same Cavalcanti Ono

ID: 30.291.088

Shohreh Taghavaeearaby
ID: 3.306.696
Sonia Banaki Sanches
ID: 3.306.696

Patient:

RG:

APPENDIX 2: Evaluation Form

Name: ____

Age:years Date of birth: /_____________________/ Sex: ( )Female ( )Male

Address:City:

E-mail:Mobile:Telephone:

Responsible person's name:Responsible person's telephone number:

QUESTIONNAIRE:

1) How long ago were you diagnosed with Parkinson's disease?years.

2) Do you take any medication for Parkinson's disease?

( ) Yes ( ) No. Which ones?

3) Are you taking any alternative treatments for Parkinson's?

( ) Yes ( ) No. Which ones?

4) Do you have any family members diagnosed with Parkinson's disease?

( )Yes ( )No. Who?

5) Do you have any other pathologies already diagnosed?

( ) Yes ( ) No. Which ones?

6) Are you undergoing treatment for other conditions?

( ) Yes ( ) No. Which ones?

7) Do you take any medication for other conditions?

( ) Yes ( ) No. Which ones?

8) Do you currently practise any physical activity? ( ) Yes ( ) No.

9) What activity do you practise?

10) How many times a week do you practise?

11) How long will the activity last?

12) Was the physical activity you do on medical advice? ( )Yes ( )No.

13) Is the physical activity you do enjoyable? ( )Yes ( )No.

14) Have you ever had a professional massage?

( ) Yes ( ) No. Which?

15) Before the diagnosis of the disease? ( )Yes ( )No.

16) For what purpose?

17) Did you like the result: ( ) Yes ( ) No.

18) What can you expect from the massages you'll receive during the research? What are your

expectations?

19)   Main symptoms:

( )Sleep disorders

( )Muscle stiffness

( )Tremors

( )Depression

( )Constipation

( )Tiredness

( )Non-specific pains

( )Speech difficulties

( )Difficulty swallowing

( )Other. Which?

- IN RELATION TO YOUR SLEEP:

20)   Do you sleep well? ( ) Yes ( ) No.

21)   Does it take you long to fall asleep? ( ) Yes ( ) No.

22)   Do you wake up at night? ( ) Yes ( ) No.

23)   How many hours do you sleep a day?

24)   What time do you usually wake up?

25)   In your own words, what's your sleep like?

- IN RELATION TO MUSCLE STIFFNESS:

26)   Do you have difficulty making any movements? ( ) Yes ( ) No.

27)   Where on the body?

28)   Which type of movement do you find most difficult?

- IN RELATION TO TREMORS:

29)   Do you have tremors? ( ) Yes ( ) No.

30)   How did you notice his tremors?

31)   Does the tremor make it impossible for you to do anything?

( ) Yes ( ) No. Which ones?

32)   Which parts of the body are most affected by tremors?

- IN RELATION TO DEPRESSION:

33)   Do you get angry easily? ( )Yes ( )No.

34)   Do you feel stressed? ( ) Yes ( ) No.

35)   Do you feel discouraged? ( ) Yes ( ) No.

36)   Do you consider yourself an optimistic person? ( ) Yes ( ) No.

37)   Do you get on well with your family? ( ) Yes ( ) No.

38)   Do you get on well with other people in your social life? ( ) Yes ( ) No

39)   How do you deal with everyday problems?

40)   Do you have faith? ( ) Yes ( ) No.

41) What do you believe?

- IN RELATION TO CONSTIPATION:

42) How often do you have a bowel movement?

43) Do you have difficulty evacuating? ( ) Yes ( ) No.

44) Do you feel pain when you defecate? ( ) Yes ( ) No.

45) Do you take a long time to evacuate? ( ) Yes ( ) No.

46) Do you drink a lot of fluids? ( ) Yes ( ) No.

47) Do you take any kind of medication to pass bowel movements?

( ) Yes ( ) No. Which ones?

- IN RELATION TO TIREDNESS:

48) Do you get tired easily? ( ) Yes ( ) No.

49) Does tiredness get in the way of carrying out your activities? ( ) Yes ( ) No.

50) Which activities are hampered by tiredness?

51) When do you feel most tired?

- IN RELATION TO NON-SPECIFIC PAIN:

52) Do you usually feel any kind of pain? ( ) Yes ( ) No.

53) Does it get in the way of your daily activities? ( ) Yes ( ) No.

54) Where does the pain occur?

55) When do the pains occur?

56) How often do they occur?

- IN RELATION TO SPEECH ALTERATIONS:

57) Have you noticed any changes in your speech? ( ) Yes ( ) No.

58) Do you think your speech has become slurred? ( ) Yes ( ) No.

59) Do you think your speech has slowed down? ( ) Yes ( ) No.

- IN RELATION TO DIFFICULTY SWALLOWING:

60) Do you currently have any difficulty chewing? ( ) Yes ( ) No.

61) Do you find it difficult to swallow? ( )Yes ( )No.

62) Do you choke easily? ( ) Yes ( ) No.

63) Have there been any changes in your eating habits since Parkinson's?

( ) Yes ( ) No. Which ones?

64) How many meals do you eat a day?

I declare that the information I have provided is true.

Londrina, 2017.

Signature:.

Patient:Date: ____ //

Therapist: ____

- QUALITY OF SLEEP:

Ótimo   Bom   Regular   Ruim   Péssimo

- MUSCLE RIGIDITY:

Ótimo   Bom   Regular   Ruim   Péssimo

- TREMORS:

Ótimo   Bom   Regular   Ruim   Péssimo

- TRISTEZA:

Ótimo   Bom   Regular   Ruim   Péssimo

- CONSTIPATION

Ótimo   Bom   Regular   Ruim   Péssimo

- TIRED:

Ótimo   Bom   Regular   Ruim   Péssimo

- NON-SPECIFIC PAIN:

Ótimo   Bom   Regular   Ruim   Péssimo

- SPEECH DIFFICULTIES:

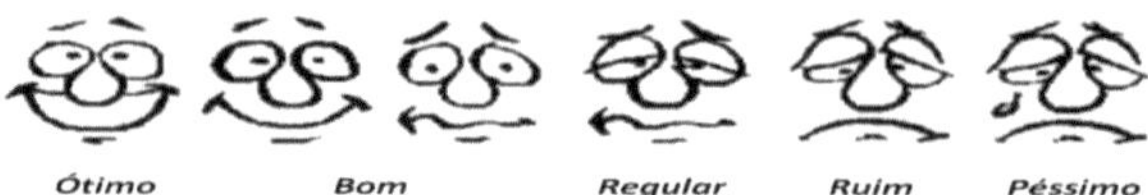

- DIFFICULTY SWALLOWING:

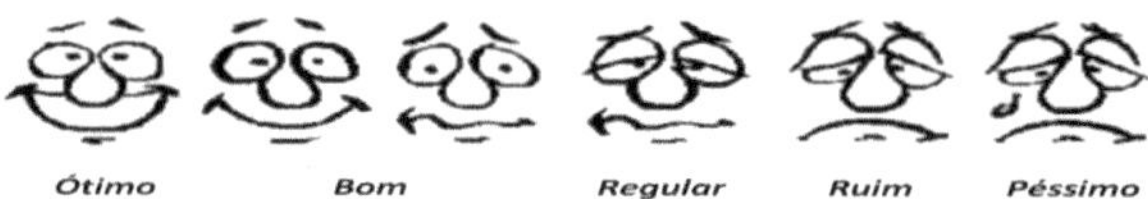

- RELAXATION:

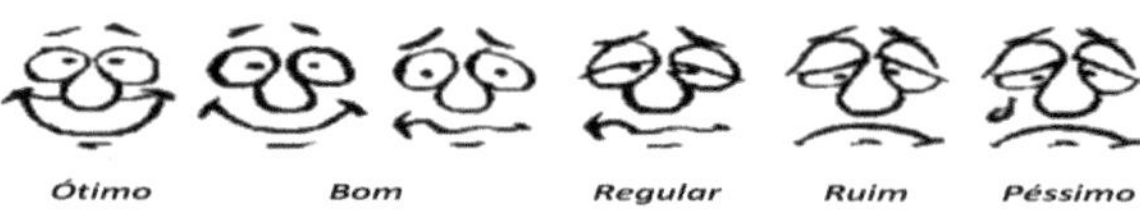

- WHAT YOUR DAYS WERE LIKE:

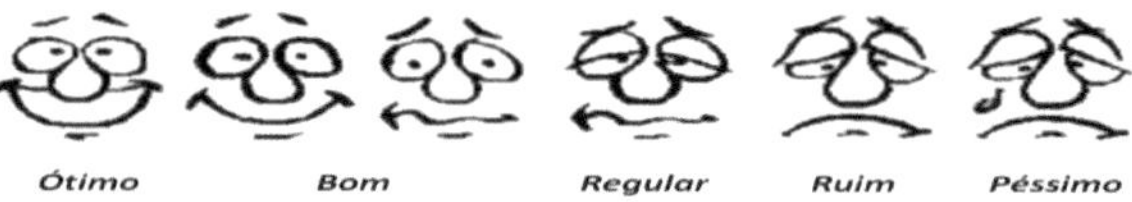

MARK WHERE YOU FEEL THE MOST PAIN:

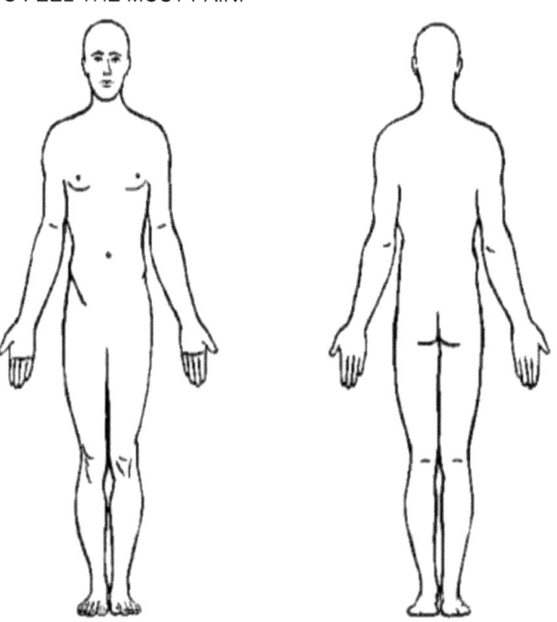

HAS ANYTHING DIFFERENT HAPPENED THIS WEEK?

____
____
____
____
____
____
____
____
____
____
____
____

EXCLUSIVE FIELD FOR MASSAGE THERAPISTS:

Did the patient sleep? ( )Yes ( )No

Was the patient able to relax? ( )Yes ( )No

Was there a reduction in tremors? ( )Yes ( )No

Was there a reduction in pain? ( )Yes ( )No

Notes:

____
____
____
____
____
____
____
____
____
____
____
____
____
____
____
____
____
____
____
____
____
____

Patient:Therapist:

APPENDIX 4: Conclusion Form

Patient:Date: ____ //

Therapist: _______________________________________

1) Do you currently work? ( )Yes ( )No

2) Are you retired? ( )Yes ( )No

3) Are you married? ( )Yes ( )No

4) Do you live alone? ( )Yes ( )No

5) Do you have children? ( )Yes ( )No

6) Do you have grandchildren? ( )Yes ( )No

7) Do you have a good relationship with your family? ( )Yes ( )No

8) Do you often have nightmares or troubled dreams? ( )Yes ( )No

9) When you started receiving care, did you believe in a positive outcome? ( )Yes ( )No

10) Would you continue treatment if it were possible? ( )Yes ( )No

11) Do you intend to continue the massage treatment after the project?

( )Yes ( )No

12) Would you recommend massage to another Parkinson's sufferer?

13) Did you notice any physical changes during the time you received the massage? ( )Yes ( )No

14) Did you notice any emotional changes during the treatment period?

( )Yes ( )No

15) Did your family notice any changes in you during the time you took part in the project? ( )Yes ( )No

16) Now that you've learnt about massage therapy, how do you see it?

17) What is your assessment of the project?

18) What is your assessment of the service?

19) What was it like for you to take part in the project?

20) Give a positive review.

21) Make a negative criticism.

APPENDIX 5: Sequence of Manoeuvres Performed

a) PRONE POSITION

BACK (20 minutes)

- Shallow and deep glides with both hands flat on the entire back;
- Slide with alternating hands and two thumbs on the paravertebral region;
- Compression with the knuckles on the paravertebral muscles and the scapula region;
- Rolling of the paravertebrals;
- Kneading on the trapezius and sliding from the neck to the shoulders;
- Slide with the lateral edge of the hands from the trapezius to the cervical region;
- Friction with the thumbs all over the spine;

- Sliding in the lumbar region, from the centre to the waist;
- Tapotage of the entire back;

THIGH (5 minutes)
- Shallow and deep glides with the hands flat on the entire thigh;
- Sliding with alternating hands;
- Sliding with both hands in a transverse direction (twisting);
- Alternate glides with the thumb across the thigh;
- Circular pressure movements with the thumb;
- Kneading with thumb and fingers;
- Superficial sliding on the entire thigh;
- Quadriceps stretching.

LEG (5 minutes)
- Shallow and deep glides with the hands flat on the entire leg;
- Sliding with alternating hands;
- Sliding with both hands in a transverse direction (twisting);
- Alternate slides with the thumb down the entire leg;
- Circular pressure movements with the thumb;
- Kneading with thumb and fingers;
- Surface slippage.

b) SUPINE POSITION

FOOT MASSAGE (10 minutes)
- Alternating shallow sliding with the thumbs, on the sole of the foot.
- Circular movements with the thumb on the lateral and medial edge;
- Slide your knuckles with closed hands on the sole of your foot;
- Kneading of the heel and heel tendon;
- Slip in the dorsal region of the foot, towards the ankle;
- Circular sliding on the malleoli;
- Slipping on the toes;
- Circular joint movement in each finger;
- Passive foot mobilisations;
- Stretching.

LEG (4 minutes)
- Shallow and deep glides with the hands flat on the entire leg;

- Sliding with alternating hands;
- Sliding with both hands in a transverse direction (twisting);
- Alternate slides with the thumb down the entire leg;
- Superficial sliding on the whole leg;

THIGH (4 minutes)

- Shallow and deep glides with the hands flat on the entire thigh;
- Sliding with alternating hands;
- Sliding with both hands in a transverse direction (twisting);
- Alternate glides with the thumb across the thigh;
- Circular pressure movements with the thumb;
- Kneading with thumb and fingers;
- Circular movements with your fingertips around the entire patella.
- Passive hip circumduction mobilisations to both sides;
- Hamstring and sural triceps stretches;
- Superficial sliding on the entire thigh;

ABDOME (4 minutes)

- Superficial sliding of the xiphoid process, encircling the ribs and ending in the rectus abdominis fibre;
- Superficial and then deep clockwise sliding of the entire abdominal area;
- Kneading of the abdomen;
- Wave motion with the palms of the hands;
- Circular rubbing around the navel;
- Superficial sliding of the xiphoid process, encircling the ribs and ending in the rectus abdominis fibre;

ARM (4 minutes)

- Shallow and deep glides with the hands flat on the entire arm;
- Sliding with alternating hands;
- Sliding with both hands in a transverse direction (twisting);
- Alternate glides with the thumb along the entire arm;
- Circular pressure movements with the thumb;
- Kneading with thumb and fingers;
- Superficial sliding on the whole arm;
- Sliding around the shoulder.

ANTEBRACH (4 minutes)

- Shallow and deep glides with the hands flat on the entire arm;
- Sliding with alternating hands;
- Sliding with both hands in a transverse direction (twisting);
- Alternate glides with the thumb along the entire arm;
- Circular pressure movements with the thumb;
- Kneading with thumb and fingers;
- Superficial sliding on the whole arm;

HANDS (5 minutes)
- Circular movements over the entire palmar region;
- Alternate sliding with the thumb;
- Sliding with the palms of your hands;
- Sliding, circumduction and traction movements on all fingers;
- Wrist joint movements: flexion, extension and circumduction;
- Slippage of the dorsal region of the hand;
- Sliding in the entire upper limbs.

HEAD AND FACE (5 minutes)
- Slide from the sternum, over the shoulders and along the trapezius;
- Friction and compression with the thumb on points of the trapezius;
- Sliding in the entire cervical region;
- Friction with the fingers in the occipital region; temporal, parietal;
- Mobilising the ears with circular movements and rubbing;
- Simultaneous and alternating sliding of the jaw towards the ears;
- Sliding of the frontal region towards the ears;
- Friction with the fingers in the frontal, temporal, parietal and occipital regions;
- Slide your thumbs over the eyebrows and around the eye sockets.
- Tweezing and circular movements on the eyebrows;
- Glide your fingertips over your cheekbones;
- Glide over the entire face;
- Cervical traction;
- Stretching the trapezius;
- ECOM and trapezius stretching;
- Laying hands on the face.

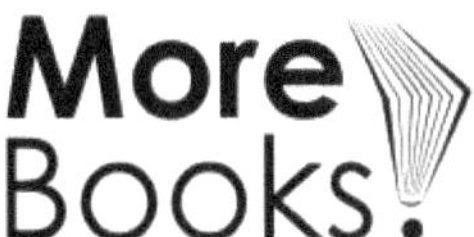

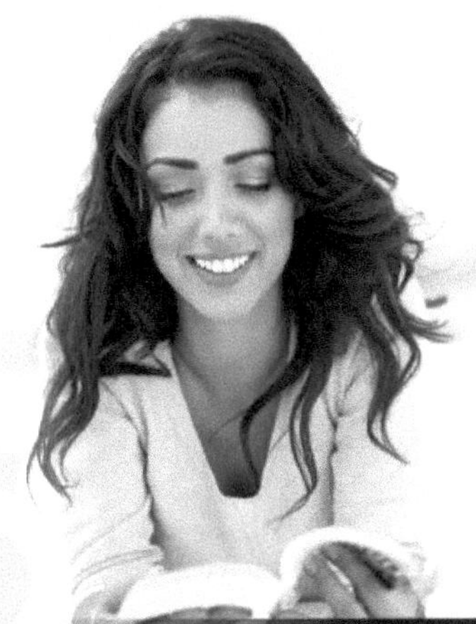

I want morebooks!

Buy your books fast and straightforward online - at one of world's fastest growing online book stores! Environmentally sound due to Print-on-Demand technologies.

Buy your books online at
www.morebooks.shop

Kaufen Sie Ihre Bücher schnell und unkompliziert online – auf einer der am schnellsten wachsenden Buchhandelsplattformen weltweit! Dank Print-On-Demand umwelt- und ressourcenschonend produziert.

Bücher schneller online kaufen
www.morebooks.shop

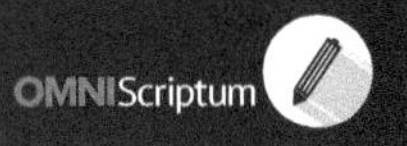

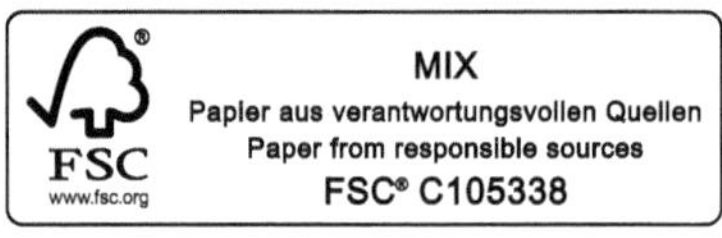

Printed by Books on Demand GmbH, Norderstedt / Germany